An Easy Way To Understand Crohn's Disease and IBD

Brian B Jacques.

Part of a Series of Mini Health Books

Wisdom For Life Media

Publisher: Wisdom For Life Media

While they have made every effort to verify the information provided in this book, neither the author nor the publisher assumes any responsibility for errors in, omissions from, or different interpretation of the subject matter.

The information herein may be subject to varying laws, regulations, and practices in different areas, states and countries. The purchaser or reader assumes all responsibility for use of the information.

All information included within this book is for educational purposes only. The author and publishers do not attempt to diagnose or treat any medical conditions, be it to do with health, diet or exercise.

If you consider that you have any kind of medical condition, then, you should consult a qualified medical practitioner or doctor before starting any vitamin and/or mineral program or supplement regime, exercise or health training program or diet suggested in this book.

This book is not intended for anyone under the age of 18 years, nor is it intended for breast feeding or pregnant women, underweight people or anyone with eating disorders or a health condition that requires special diets or medical treatment.

The author and publishers disclaim any liability for any loss however caused by anyone using the information contained in this book.

ISBN-13: 978-1500784881

ISBN-10: 1500784885

Contents

4   Brian B Jacques.

Chapter 1

A Brief Description of Crohn's Disease

Let me start by giving you a brief description of Crohn's disease–what it is and how it affects you. Crohn's disease was renamed in 1932 from ileitis. It was named after Burrill Bernard Crohn It is basically a multifaceted condition that affects your entire digestive tract, all the way from the mouth to the anus. It is characterized by ulcers and inflammation. The most common area affected is the small and large intestines, but other organs can be affected too.

The symptoms of Crohn's disease come and go during your lifetime. It is called remission when the symptoms appear to have disappeared and relapse when they suddenly reappear again. Doctors can suggest and prescribe different medications which are designed to help control abdominal cramping, inflammation and pain caused by the disease.

At the present time, there is no cure for Crohn's disease, and it is not known what causes it. I am sure that at some point in the future, scientists will be able to determine a cause and then they will be able to work on a control protocol or possibly a cure.

With the onset of Crohn's disease, shallow erosions usually appear in the intestinal walls. The inflammatory response increases as the disease develops which increases the size and depth of the intestinal wall erosions which then leads to an ulcerated condition.

Work done so far by researchers suggests the cause could be more biological than emotional. So individuals with certain personality types are no more likely to develop Crohn's disease than anyone else. Certain theories have been suggested including an autoimmune condition or bacterial infection, even low stomach acid–which can be an issue as a person ages, but to date there is no definitive answer as to what causes Crohn's disease.

Individuals who suffer from Crohn's disease will have various symptoms including: abdominal pain, diarrhea or constipation, fever, fistulas, loss of appetite, possible obstructions, ulcerations and weight loss–which is caused by the malabsorption of nutrients from food, due to the small intestine being compromised.

The intestines may empty frequently due to the pain and swelling in the intestines; this in turn can cause cramping and pain as well as bleeding around the anus. Your doctor will use barium enemas and do an x ray of the small intestine in addition to performing a colonoscopy to determine what problems your Crohn's disease is causing. Once a definitive diagnosis has been made, your doctor will suggest identifying foods that cause irritation, and then eliminate them from your diet.

It might be advisable to try an elimination diet to start with. Usually rice and pears are fairly safe, and then reintroduce foods one at a time to see if you have a reaction to them. If you do, then you will know to leave them out of your diet. Additionally, your doctor can prescribe certain medications to suppress the immune system or ease the inflammation. These medications may include steroids or antibiotics; in addition, surgery may be necessary.

To sum up, Crohn's disease is a complex and varied issue. It is not understood at this time what causes this condition, or why it goes into remission and then reappears. The symptoms are as described above and doctors continue to strive to find a cure or a better way to control this very distressing disease.

Chapter 2

Inflammatory Bowel Disease

What is inflammatory bowel disease and how does it affect you? Basically it is a disease that affects the digestive system. The digestive system extends all the way from the mouth to the anus. Interestingly this system is full of germs and bacteria.

The "good" bacteria are used by the body to break down food ready for absorption through the small intestine. The majority of this activity should be performed by enzymes from the raw food that we consume. Unfortunately this does not always happen. This is due in part to the high amounts of saturated fats, sugars, salt, additives and processed foods which make up the major part of the Western diet.

This type of diet increases the fermentation process in the intestines. So, whether by fermentation or the actions of enzymes, "good" bacteria play a critical role in the food digestion process. One problem arises when you take a course of antibiotics.

Antibiotics take no prisoners. They not only kill the infection–which they are designed to do–but they also kill all the good bacteria as well. This is why people often have a bout of diarrhea when taking antibiotics. This is due to the death of friendly bacteria in the intestines. In fact it is a good idea to take a course of probiotics–which can be in the form of yogurt or as a capsule supplement to help the body replace these friendly bacteria.

Therefore, when we talk about inflammatory bowel disease, we are dealing with a disease of the digestive tract. This disease usually causes problems for most individuals in the small or large intestines. But bear in mind that it can also occur elsewhere as well. This disease is defined as either ulcerative colitis or Crohn's disease. Both of these conditions have a marked effect on how the intestines convert the food we eat and then how the nutrients from the food are absorbed into the body.

There are no exact numbers available for how many Americans have inflammatory bowel disease. Estimates put the figure at between 1 and 2 million. The majority are diagnosed between the ages of 20–30, but younger children and older adults can be diagnosed too.

The number of cases diagnosed is higher in Western cultures than in Asian cultures. This is due in part to the Western diet which as described above, is high in saturated fat, sugar and salt, etc. Research to date points to the disease being more of a biological factor, rather than an emotional or personality one. But there is no conclusive proof either way.

Many people confuse inflammatory bowel disease with irritable bowel syndrome. But they are totally different. With irritable bowel syndrome there is no change in the integrity of the intestines–either physically or biologically. It is caused more by stress and emotional changes than anything else. By reducing stress levels and compensating for any emotional changes, individuals with this condition can significantly reduce its effects.

By comparison, inflammatory bowel disease is far more serious. Of the two, ulcerative colitis produces fewer side effects. It does not penetrate as far into the intestinal wall as Crohn's disease does; and is more frequently found in the rectal area where it causes frequent diarrhea.

Crohn's disease on the other hand is often in the lower end of the small intestines–but bear in mind it is not always limited to just this area. It penetrates further into the intestinal wall than ulcerative colitis and as a result causes ulceration and inflammation.

There is no definitive answer as to what causes inflammatory bowel disease. Researchers theorize that it could be to do with diet, environmental issues or hereditary factors.

The most frequent symptoms of inflammatory bowel disease are abdominal pain and diarrhea. If the diarrhea is excessive, it can cause dehydration as well as leading to bleeding in the large intestine caused by the irritation and inflammation. In consequence, there will be an increase in the heart rate caused by dehydration as well as a drop in blood pressure. If the bleeding continues, this can cause anemia and a drop in the red blood cell count.

To sum up, inflammatory bowel disease is an important medical and social problem, but with correct medical care and diet and lifestyle changes, individuals can lead a beneficial and worthwhile life.

Chapter 3

Crohn's Disease and IBD Risk factors

Whilst there is no definite reason why Inflammatory Bowel Disease (IBD) will develop, researchers have various theories and have assessed several risk factors for Crohn's disease and IBD.

In a previous chapter, I mentioned several possible causes: autoimmune concerns, bacterial infections and low stomach acid. Researchers from Massachusetts General Hospital have more recently identified various genetic factors which are linked to Crohn's disease. These new discoveries can potentially lead to new forms of treatment for this disease.

In identifying genetic factors, it has been ascertained that Crohn's disease often runs in families with the instances varying between sex, age and residential location. Incidentally, Crohn's disease is identified to be the second most commonly diagnosed inflammatory disease after rheumatoid arthritis.

There is no distinction that more men will develop Crohn's disease than women–in fact it affects men and women equally. Interestingly, it appears to affect the Jewish population more and Black Americans less than other ethnic groups. Between ages 20-30 appears to be the main age range where Crohn's disease is diagnosed. However children can be diagnosed with the disease in addition to older adults–especially between ages 50-80.

An additional risk factor appears to be if you live in a city as opposed to living in the country. Additionally highly developed Western countries seem to have a higher risk factor than nations that are less developed. All of this suggests that it is not only genetics that plays a role, but diet and environmental considerations do as well.

While various risk factors for Crohn's disease and IBD have been identified, the exact causes why someone will develop this disease remains as elusive as ever. It seems the decreased number of people diagnosed in less developed countries may lead researchers to focus on diet and lifestyle considerations, which may have a bearing on determining how to improve the body's ability to go into remission. This will potentially alleviate the unpleasant symptoms that a person can experience, and as an added benefit, the large and small intestines will not become so impaired.

Chapter 4

Psychology and Inflammatory Bowel Disease

An individual's personal psychology has no link to the cause of inflammatory bowel disease. But research suggests that stress and anxiety can change the severity of the condition. What this means is that being under stress or anxious will not contribute to someone developing inflammatory bowel disease. But what it does mean is that someone who is already suffering from the condition will experience increased symptoms. Some 50 years ago it was thought that specific personality types were at risk of developing certain types of illnesses. However, research has found that IBD is purely biologically based.

Different individuals deal with different situations in different ways; in particular those situations that have a major impact on what they do each day. Health issues can present a special challenge as they not only affect quality of life but have an impact on family, physical and emotional issues as well. Emotional issues can include feelings of guilt, depression and even denial of the condition. Even the need that help is required may be a denial condition as well. When these situations arise–that affect relationships with others it is time to seek help from a qualified and licensed therapist.

It has sometimes been the case that the family of an inflammatory bowel disease sufferer blame themselves for their family members condition–especially where the disease involves their children or spouse. But remember, the disease is biological in nature and is not transmitted from person to person.

Doing a planning session before leaving home can alleviate any worries or anxiety concerning possible personal accidents or embarrassing situations. Having knowledge of where the restrooms are before sitting down in a restaurant or going on a shopping expedition to the local mall will make you feel more comfortable and relaxed.

It is also a good idea to take extra clothing and sanitary protection with you in case it is needed. Don't try and hide the fact that you have a health condition from those close to you. If you are up front about your inflammatory bowel condition, then those around you will feel more at ease too.

It is important to listen to your body and understand what foods can cause flare-ups, and then avoid those foods. If you can give your intestines an easy life then they will reward you with less pain and discomfort as well as less intestinal damage for you to cope with.

Chapter 5

Crohn's Disease and Pain Management

When managing pain for Crohn's disease, you will have to determine the type of pain you are trying to alleviate. Pain associated with Crohn's disease is usually in the abdominal area and involves cramping as well as back pain.

Imagine pain associated with Crohn's disease. You can liken it to stomach flu where you continually vomit or feel nauseated and have diarrhea and stomach cramps for 24 hours each day. You cannot keep food or drink down–or hardly so, and your stomach feels so sore as if someone has punched you. You are experiencing a low grade fever and you have aches in every joint in your body. Now just try and imagine having those symptoms for many weeks at a time when your Crohn's disease goes into relapse.

And as I explained previously–to really make your day–there is no known cure for Crohn's disease–and the real cause is not known either. Your doctor can prescribe certain medications to relieve the pain–but these are rather limited in their result. There are also certain natural remedies that you can try. I cover natural remedies later in this book.

The goal is to get your Crohn's disease into remission. But sometimes this is not possible and surgery is the only alternative, to remove part of the bowel that is so diseased or swollen that it restricts the uptake of nutrients.

Surveys conducted with physicians around the United States found that they generally agree on the methodology to diagnose if Crohn's disease is responsible for bowel inflammation and ulceration. Where they do differ however, is in their method of treatment.

What this means is that treatment methods for Crohn's disease can vary from doctor to doctor and state to state, as well as city to city. This goes to show that with this particular disease there is no standard treatment protocol, and there are no black and white answers.

Now that you have this knowledge, and you have been diagnosed with Crohn's disease, you can now consult different physicians if you feel the treatment you are currently receiving is not being adequate for your needs. Remember Crohn's disease flares up and goes into remission. If this happens though it does not necessarily mean that your current physician is not giving you the best care possible within his particular regime.

Consulting a pain management clinic is the best pathway to obtain relief from Crohn's disease. When visiting the pain management clinic the doctor's primary concern is to relieve your pain and not to locate the source of the pain or to get you back into remission. Often where Crohn's disease is involved the line gets blurred between pain management and treatment. In these cases it is the pain management part that tends to take a back seat in the general scheme of things.

One thing that pain management clinics are good at is finding suitable medications, biofeedback, various stress and anxiety management techniques in addition to different alternative therapies that will alleviate your pain.

It is important to remember that your gastroenterologist concentrates on providing treatment for ulcerations and potential obstructions. Doctors at the pain management clinic can provide daily relief for abdominal cramping and back pain.

Chapter 6

Kids and Crohn's Disease

Children who are diagnosed with Crohn's disease can experience real problems. Imagine this! Kids in the age range of 12-19 are trying to figure out who they are. They have issues with teasing, attraction to the opposite sex and hormone issues. During adolescence and puberty there is a growing body and acne to contend with as well as strange sensations and confusing thoughts and feelings. Then toss into the mix cramps, daily stomach pains and diarrhea with constant running to the bathroom.

It is therefore no wonder that kids who are diagnosed with any inflammatory bowel disease can be very picky eaters in relation to other children, and they often have more psychological problems than other teens. Of note is the increasing realization that our diets make a significant contribution to the added risk of kids developing Crohn's disease.

The standard protocol that doctors use when treating kids with Crohn's disease is to use medications that keep the inflammation in check. Steroids are often used which can lead to excessive thirst, a puffy face, a proliferation of acne and excessive weight gain. If all this is not bad enough, then some children may need surgery if there is a blockage in their intestines, or they develop a fissure or fistula.

Just as in adults, kids have the same malabsorption issues in that nutrients are often not able to be taken up through the small intestine into the body. Several important factors now come into play here, as the lack of certain vitamins and minerals in a child's younger growing years can lead to the development of various diseases or conditions as the child grows older. For instance, an inability to absorb the mineral calcium in the young growing years can lead to an increased incidence of osteoporosis in later life.

Other issues that can arise in kids with Crohn's disease are an inability to interact with other children, an increased incidence of teasing, social issues, behavioral problems and possibly family dysfunction.

Researchers have discovered that kids with Crohn's disease thrive in a support group with other kids who have the same condition. Additionally, children also respond well where there is structure within a family with regard to meal habits and encouragement in projecting a good body image.

As with adults, certain foods will cause pain in kids; but this tends to be more of an individual thing. Research shows that a particular food may affect your son or daughter, but it may not affect another person's son or daughter who also has inflammatory bowel disease.

Both children and parents have a challenging time on their hands when it is the kids who have been diagnosed with Crohn's disease. However, kids who have supportive parents and attend support groups tend to do better at school then those kids who do not have these advantages.

Chapter 7

Crohn's Disease and Intestinal Damage

Crohn's disease commonly affects the intestinal tract. This is where such conditions as watery diarrhea can occur. In addition, the colon can produce diarrhea mixed with blood and pus or mucus, and all this can lead the colon to inform the individual that they need an urgent bowel movement. Plus abdominal cramping may occur along with vomiting or a feeling of nausea. Also involved are loss of appetite and as a result–weight loss, as well as protracted growth.

Also the anus may become painful, sore and bleed with each bowel movement, so it is understandable with all these situations that the individual may lose their appetite and as a result lose weight. The psychological feeling would be to want to avoid bowel movements as much as possible.

As each individual is different, intestinal disease can be minimal or extensive. In the early stages of Crohn's disease, small shallow attrition may occur in the inner lining of the bowel. These erosions are called aphthous ulcers. Over time these ulcers spread and become larger and deeper. Ultimately this inflammatory response totally compromises the intestinal wall to the extent that they become true ulcerations.

The body tries its best to heal the ulceration, but in so doing, the bowel becomes narrower and stiffens. In time this can lead to an obstruction which can build up gradually, or can happen suddenly requiring immediate surgery. When an obstruction occurs, food that has been digested as well as fluids and gas cannot pass through into the colon. Obstructions in the small intestinal can lead to cramping, distention, nausea and vomiting.

Of more serious concern, Crohn's disease can progress to the extent that it can perforate the intestinal wall which will lead to bowel fluid leaking into the abdominal cavity. This in turn will infect adjacent organs causing peritonitis which is life threatening.

A tunnel can be created between the intestine and adjacent organ should an ulcer penetrate through the intestinal wall. An abdominal abscess is formed if the tunnel reaches a space. A fistula is formed if the tunnel reaches an organ. Fistulas are most frequently formed between the intestines and bladder, anus, skin and vagina.

While I have described some of the more dramatic events that can happen in the intestines, more insidious events can occur involving the lack of uptake of nutrients through the small intestine from the food you eat. This is due to the damage caused to the small intestinal wall by the Crohn's disease. Even though the individual can eat a good normal healthy diet they can become malnourished. And where bleeding develops around the anus and / or in the intestines a person can become anemic, experience a low red blood cell count all of which can lead to fatigue, a pale skin and shortness of breath.

Of major concern, due to the significant changes in the structure of the intestinal walls caused by the Crohn's disease, sufferers become more at risk of developing colon cancer years after the inception of the disease.

Chapter 8

Bacteria and Crohn's Disease

As mentioned earlier, researchers and scientists have theorized that bacteria may be one of the contributory factors in a person developing Crohn's disease.

To date, doctors and microbiologists have been unable to culture specific bacteria in the blood of patients with Crohn's disease. However, a bacterium has been identified: Mycobacterium avium subspecies paratuberculosis (or MAP). Molecular biologists at the University of Central Florida identified MAP within the blood of half the patients diagnosed with Crohn's disease, and none in the blood of people who are healthy.

Leprosy and tuberculosis is in the same class of microbes as MAP. The bacteria resides in cell walls of the infected person, but does not cause cell damage, neither does it have known toxins. But damage is caused by the infected person's body reaction to the bacteria. MAP causes an immune reaction to be triggered against the body's own tissue (much like an autoimmune response) where MAP is hiding primarily in the gut walls.

MAP cells can demonstrate amazing abilities: they are able to shed there own cell walls (without a cell wall they are called sphereoblasts) and quietly exist in a condition that is hard to detect under a light microscope. They can lie dormant in this way for many years and then suddenly grow new cell walls and become active once more.

Of note–when bacteria are present in the blood it is deemed to be systemic; in other words–a bacterial infection that is present throughout the entire body. Data that is available on MAP does not suggest that it is systemic, but is more like an onlooker. This in turn can raise a very important question which needs further investigation. The question is: did the Crohn's disease come before the bacteria, or vice versa. The answer to this important question could have a profound effect on developing a preventative program and treatment protocol for Crohn's disease.

MAP bacterium is not limited to humans. It is also responsible for Johne's disease–a very similar intestinal disease which is found in cattle, goats and sheep. As there is a link here between animals and humans, researchers theorize that there may be a transition here through milk or meat, or both. Although milk is pasteurized, according to one research scientist, MAP bacterium was found in four samples of whole pasteurized milk bought randomly from retail outlets. As a result there is some concern that a pasteurization process may not be as effective as it should be.

To date MAP has been identified in several states and other countries including: California, Texas, Australia and France–but the information is rather scarce. It has proved difficult to isolate MAP from other bacteria in the gut due to its ability to shed its protective cell wall. The usual method is for scientists to kill off the unwanted bacteria and try and keep the one they want to study. But as just explained this is proving rather difficult with MAP as the shedding of the cell wall can also kill the MAP.

As an ongoing research project, it is encouraging to see that a bacteria has been identified that potentially can be used to find a treatment and medication program to alleviate this very distressing disease.

Chapter 9

Crohn's Disease and Low Stomach Acid

Adults and children can be affected by several inflammatory bowel diseases–and Crohn's disease is one of them. Inflammatory bowel disease appears to be on the increase as the nutritional value of the food we eat decreases and at the same time, stress levels are on the increase. Is there a correlation between the two?

Researchers have discovered that in diet studies, people who consume more sugar and less raw fruit and vegetables have a greater risk of developing Crohn's disease than those people who consume less sugar and eat more raw fruit and vegetables.

There is a distinct linkage between Crohn's disease and low stomach acid. As stated previously, Crohn's disease and the inflammation, pain and cramping that is associated with it, are all linked to the large and small intestines. Therefore it would be safe to assume, that if the level of stomach acid was reduced, then the level of inflammation and pain would also reduce as would other side effects of the disease.

The majority of physicians know that the health of the stomach is intimately linked to the health of the large and small intestines. Of note! Where Crohn's disease or ulcerative colitis is present, there appears to be a lower incidence of gastric activity than would normally be the case. This has been confirmed by medical testing.

What is interesting is the statement in the previous paragraph. In reality the opposite is true. The lower the stomach acid the body produces, the more likely the individual is to develop an inflammatory condition in the lower intestine and colon. This inflammatory condition can take various forms including: Crohn's disease, Irritable Bowel Syndrome, inflammatory bowel disease or Ulcerative colitis.

Low stomach acid can be the result of various issues. Age is one of them. As a person ages, they tend to produce less stomach acid. Another issue is directly linked to the "Western Diet". This tends to be high in sugar, sodium (salt) and saturated fat. In addition there is a high consumption of red meat. All of this can lead to an increased risk of developing an inflammatory bowel illness and an over-growth of unfriendly bacteria in the gut.

Enzymes play a critical role in the digestion of our food. The body produces certain enzymes, and others are contained within the food itself. Enzymes are the body's workers–they make things happen. And each enzyme plays a specific role in the digestive process. For instance, an enzyme whose purpose is to digest proteins won't digest fiber or starches. And conversely, an enzyme whose purpose is to break down fiber and starches won't break down proteins. Unfortunately with the high amount of red meat and sugar consumed in the average diet, the digestive process has become more fermentative. This is evidenced by changes in stomach acid production, and the disruption of bacterial flora in feces.

If you have been diagnosed with Crohn's disease it is prudent to eliminate or at least reduce your consumption of red meat and dairy products. This will help reduce inflammation and increase the production of stomach acid. As explained previously, a low stomach acid condition is a risk factor for developing an inflammatory condition in the intestinal tract. This can be kept under control by consuming well balanced nutritious meals and eliminating where possible any processed foods which contain artificial ingredients and are high in saturated fat, sugar, sodium (salt) and sugar.

By following some of the recommendation outlined in this chapter, you can give your body a big boost to heal itself. In the short term, medications can help bring your Crohn's disease under control. But it is only through your intervention and changes you adopt in your diet and lifestyle, that you will have any chance at all to experience an improvement in your pain and discomfort. The benefit will be pain free days, which I am sure you will agree, will improve your quality of life.

Chapter 10

Alcohol Abuse and Crohn's Disease

As Crohn's disease is an inflammatory disease that primarily affects the large and small intestine, it is often treated with steroids and corticosteroids. Mixing alcohol with these medications will put the body under a greater degree of stress which can lead to an increased risk of infection.

The combination of steroids and alcohol impairs the immune system which means that the body has a reduced ability to fight off any infection. In some cases this can lead to an excessive bacterial infection that can cause the premature death of the person.

The consumption of beer can worsen some people's symptoms of inflammatory bowel disease–and especially Crohn's disease. This can be caused by the intestinal gas that the beer causes. However, in other cases, people find that the occasional cocktail or drink of beer does not cause any adverse effect with their symptoms.

To date there have been no conclusive studies that show alcohol consumption triggers or aggravates inflammatory bowel disease and especially Crohn's disease. As mentioned in the previous paragraph–the main problem is the intestinal gas that is generated.

However, there is definite proof that the consumption of excessive alcohol can lead to arterial problems, degenerative mental capacities, liver failure (cirrhosis of the liver), gastric ulcers and a premature death.

The liver is adversely affected by alcohol consumption. Alcohol can decrease the function of the liver in addition to altering or destroying the liver's cells. One of the responsibilities of the liver is the removal of toxins. Without the support of this vital organ, your health will show a very rapid decline.

One way to support the liver–especially if you drink alcohol, is to take a Milk Thistle supplement. One of the active ingredients in Milk Thistle is silymarin which comprises three component parts: silibinin, silidianin and silicristin. Silymarin supports the liver by performing a detoxifying process and purging the effects of alcohol from liver cells. Through protein synthesis, Milk Thistle can also increase the production of new liver cells.

There are some recommendations published for alcohol consumption– and some studies show that one drink each day can help support the coronary system. One drink is defined as: 4-5 ounces of wine, 10 ounces of a wine cooler, 12 ounces of beer or 1¼ ounces of distilled liquor.

One drug (Naltrexone) that is used to treat people who consume excessive alcohol has been shown to put certain people who have Crohn's disease into remission. Naltrexone has been approved by the FDA to assist people who are going through a withdrawal process from drugs or alcohol.

Why this drugs works in cases of Crohn's disease is unclear. Researchers theorize that because the drug is an opiate, and therefore works in an inflammatory environment–and Crohn's disease is an inflammatory condition, then there might be a cell reversal of the process.

A study conducted at Penn State College of Medicine where patients took low doses of Naltrexone at night experienced minimal side effects; in fact 89 percent experienced an improvement and 67 percent had a total remission of their Crohn's disease symptoms. Currently there are two further studies in process or awaiting approval from the National Institute of Health (NIH) to do further studies on the mechanism and replicate the results.

In summary: while a small consumption of alcohol may not cause increased inflammatory symptoms, scientists know that Crohn's disease and excessive alcohol consumption has an increased negative impact on the Crohn's disease condition and also your overall health as well. And interestingly, medication used to treat the withdrawal symptoms of alcohol abuse in some cases puts Crohn's disease into a remissive state.

Chapter 11

Back Pain and Crohn's Disease

As mentioned previously, Crohn's disease causes inflammation and can also cause an obstruction in the intestines, which can lead to a blockage that restricts the uptake of nutrients from your food as well as restricting the passage of waste. These conditions can cause pain and discomfort.

Individuals, who have been diagnosed with Crohn's disease and experience back pain as well, may also be prone to osteoporosis due to years of poor absorption of nutrients and a lack of calcium.

In addition to the back pain being associated with osteoporosis, it can also be linked to digestive problems, including cramping and diarrhea, as well as fistulas or ulcers.

In order to treat Crohn's disease and back pain, the source of the back pain must first be identified. If it is linked to a digestive disorder, then working to eliminate the inflammation should clear up the back pain.

Another area that may need investigation is to determine if the back pain is originating from muscles in the back, or to muscle tension, and whether bone structure is involved–which is not linked to osteoporosis as discussed earlier. In order to alleviate this problem, it would be wise to make every effort to reduce intestinal inflammation and enhance the uptake of nutrients and at the same time, make sure that the elimination process is not hindered in any way.

Your doctor may prescribe medications to treat your Crohn's disease and back pain. These problems can be dealt with by the use of pain killers, surgical procedures in addition to dietary and lifestyle changes.

On a non-medical pathway, consulting a chiropractor has proved beneficial for many individuals who suffer from Crohn's disease and back pain. Manipulation of the spine in addition to physical therapy and massage can help alleviate many of the indications associated with inflammation of the intestines and muscle tension.

Although chiropractors do not consider that back manipulation performed by them is a cure for Crohn's disease, they do believe that it helps to ease the back pain which is linked to the Crohn's disease.

Chapter 12

Medications for Crohn's Disease

Medications fall into various categories as I have outlined below. They all have side effects, some more severe than others. It is important that you discuss your condition with your doctor so that you can work out a treatment regime that you feel comfortable with.

The various categories are:
- Aminosalicylates (5-ASAs)
- Corticosteroids (Steroids)
- Immunosuppressive Drugs
- Biologic Drugs
- Other Medications

Aminosalicylates (5-ASAs)

Aminosalicylates contain a compound 5-aminosalicylic acid, or 5-ASA, which assists in the reduction of inflammation. The purpose of these drugs is to prevent a relapse and retain a remissive state in individuals who suffer from mild to moderate Crohn's disease.

In standard form the aminosalicylate drug is **Sulfazine (Azulfidine)**. This is a combination of the 5-ASA drug **Mesalamine** and a sulfa antibiotic **Sulfapyridine**. Although the drug is effective, it comes with several side effects including: headache, nausea and rash.

Individuals who have an intolerance to **Sulfazine**, or who have an allergy to sulfa drugs can try other options of 5-ASA drugs, for example: **Mesalamine (Asacol, Pentasa)**, **Olsalazine (Dipentum)** and **Balsalazide (Colazal)**.

People with kidney disease should be cautious when taking Mesalamine as it can cause kidney problems.

Various side effects are associated with aminosalicylate drugs. Here are some of them:

- **Mesalamine** and **Balsalazide** can cause abdominal pain and cramps.
- **Mesalamine** and, **Olsalazine** can cause diarrhea.
- **Mesalamine** can cause dizziness, gas, nausea and hair loss.
- **Mesalamine** and **Balsalazide** can cause abdominal pain, cramps and headache

There appears to be no safety issues with women who are pregnant or nursing and children taking all mesalamine derivatives and sulfazine. But it is best to check with your doctor.

Corticosteroids

Corticosteroids are often referred to as steroids. They are used to treat Crohn's disease in adults due to them being very powerful anti-inflammatory drugs. As they have very serious side effects, steroids should only be used for individuals with moderate or severe Crohn's disease, or if they suffer a relapse following other drug treatments.

Women who are pregnant can safely use steroids. However, using steroids over the long term should be avoided where possible due to their side effects.

Corticosteroids are often mixed with other drugs for example, 5-ASA drugs to enhance symptom relief and quicken up withdrawal. However these combined drugs do not progress remission times.

Long term use of corticosteroids should be avoided due to serious side effects that can occur; in addition other drugs are available which have fewer side effects. Of note! Corticosteroids do not prevent flare-ups and are only used as a maintenance treatment in rare cases.

One of the problems with someone suffering from Crohn's disease is that they can become malnourished due to a lack of uptake of nutrients from the diet. In such cases these individuals are less likely to get much benefit from corticosteroids. Additionally those individuals who did not have a good initial response to corticosteroids are unlikely to do any better the second time around. Long term Crohn's disease sufferers may also build up a resistance to corticosteroids.

The most commonly prescribed corticosteroids are: **Prednisone (Deltasone), Methylprednisolone (Medrol), and Hydrocortisone (Cortef, Cortisol).** Newer corticosteroids, including **Budesonide (Entocort),** only affect localized areas in the intestine which could assist in reducing widespread side effects.

Corticosteroids can have serious and long term side effects including:

- An increased risk of infection
- Puffy facial tissue and an increase in weight
- An increased risk of acne
- Increased hair growth
- Elevated blood pressure
- Weakness in the bones with a risk of developing osteoporosis
- An increased risk of cataracts and glaucoma
- An increased risk of developing diabetes
- Muscle wasting

- An irregular menstrual cycle
- An increased risk of gastrointestinal ulcers in the upper tract.
- A change in personality. A person may become more irritable, may suffer from depression, insomnia and psychosis.

It is important to start a withdrawal program once the inflammation has subsided. Withdrawal must be done gradually otherwise if the process is done too rapidly various symptoms can occur including: fever, malaise and pain in the joints. If this happens then the dosage is increased slightly until the symptoms disappear, then the dose is reduced gradually again.

Immunosuppressive Drugs

Immunosuppressive drugs are used where it has proved difficult to control inflammatory bowel disease. They are often used for long-term treatment. They are designed to suppress the actions of the immune system, and in so doing limit the inflammatory response that is the cause of Cohn's disease. This drug class may help keep Crohn's disease in remission and also help heal fistulas and ulcers in the intestine caused by this disease. Immunosuppressive drugs are on occasions used with corticosteroids to treat a Crohn's disease flare-up.

The standard immunosuppressive drugs include **Azathioprine (Imuran, Azasan)** and **6-Mercaptopurine (6-MP, Purinethol)**. Of note! It can take from 3-6 months for these drugs to be effective. To reduce this time span, they are often combined with a low-dose corticosteroid drug. Because a lower dose is prescribed- there are fewer side effects. And as a result, the corticosteroids may be reduced at a quicker rate.

A fast acting immunosuppressant is available for individuals with severe Crohn's disease. It is called **Methotrexate (MTX, Rheumatrex, Mexate)**. It is taken on a weekly basis and is worth trying for those individuals who have tried other immunosuppressant drugs which has not worked. Be warned though! **Methotrexate** can cause liver damage as well as miscarriages and birth defects. In view of the pregnancy issues, both men and women who take **Methotrexate** should practice birth control.

There are various side effects with immunosuppressant drugs including:

- Nausea
- Vomiting
- Liver Inflammation
- Pancreatic inflammation

Individuals who also take **Cyclosporine A** or **Tacrolimus** need to have regular checks of their blood pressure and function of their kidneys.

Also, frequent tests should be done to monitor the bone marrow, as well as kidney and liver function.

Biologic Drugs

Here we have a group of genetically modified drugs that are designed to target specific proteins that are involved in inflammatory responses in the body.

According to the American Gastroenterological Association, these drugs should not be used as a prime treatment for most people with Crohn's disease. However, some individuals who have had no response after taking corticosteroids or who have fistulas may benefit from using biologic drugs as a prime treatment. But bear in mind the benefits have to be weighed up against the risks involved. Risks include: infections, lymphoma and other side effects caused by use of the drug.

Taking tumor necrosis factor (TNF) blockers, such as **Infliximab**, **Adalimumab**, and **Certolizumab**, can increase the cancer risk, especially lymphomas in children and teenagers. There is also an increased risk of developing leukemia in people of all ages.

Some individuals who have taken anti-TNF drugs have then suffered from other conditions such as psoriasis, fungal infections and tuberculosis.

It is important that your doctor carefully monitors you if you take any kind of anti-TNF therapy for any initial signs of infections. Fungal infections can include: cough, fever, malaise, shortness of breath, sweating and weight loss.

The following are a list of biologic drugs, their uses and side effects.

Infliximab (Remicade). An anti-THF-drug that is used to treat adults and children with Crohn's disease. Helps keep the disease in remission and is also used to reduce the number of fistulas and preserve closed fistulas.

Side effects include:

- Cough.
- Headache.
- Rash.
- Sinus infections and sore throat.
- Stomach pain.

Serious side effects include an increased risk of:

- Allergic reactions.
- Aplastic anemia.
- Bacterial infections.

- Fungal infections.
- Heart failure.
- Liver failure.
- Lymphoma (cancer).
- Nervous system disruption.
- Tuberculosis.
- Viral infections.

Adalimumab (Humira) is used in moderate to severe cases of Crohn's disease to stimulate a remission state in adults. It is also used to treat cases of rheumatoid arthritis. It is administered by injection which is required every two weeks.

Side effects include:

- Headache.
- Nausea.
- Rash.

Serious side effects include:

- Allergic reactions.
- Aplastic anemia.
- Bacterial infections.
- Fungal infections.
- Heart failure.
- Liver failure.
- Lymphoma (cancer).
- Nervous system disruption.
- Tuberculosis.
- Viral infections.

Note! For those individuals who carry the hepatitis B virus in their blood, this drug may restimulate it.

Certolizumab (Cimzia). This drug is prescribed to adults who have not achieved any relief with other drug programs. It is used for instances of moderate to severe Crohn's disease. Like the previous drug, it is applied by injection.

Side effects include:

* Headache.
* Nausea.
* Rash.

Serious side effects include:

- Allergic reactions.
- Aplastic anemia.
- Bacterial infections.
- Fungal infections.
- Heart failure.
- Liver failure.
- Lymphoma (cancer).
- Nervous system disruption.
- Tuberculosis.
- Viral infections.

Natalizumab (Tysabri). This drug is slightly different in that it targets white blood cells which are involved in the inflammatory response. Given by infusion, it is used to treat conditions of moderate to severe Crohn's disease.

There are some serious risks involved with this drug to the extent that individuals taking it must enroll on a special program with the FDA so that they can monitor any possible side effects associated with this drug.

Here is the most serious side effect:

- An increased risk of a rare neurological condition called progressive multifocal leukoencephalopathy (PML). This side effect is so serious that it can lead to a severe disability or even death.

Other side effects include:

- Allergic reactions.
- An increased risk of infections.
- Impaired liver function.
- Fatigue.
- Headache.
- Infusion reactions.
- Joint pain.
- Limb pain.
- Rash.
- Serious herpes infections.
- Urinary tract infections.

Note! This drug should not be used by anyone taking any form of immunosuppressant drugs.

Other Medications

Antibiotics can be used as a first case therapy for abscesses, excessive bacteria growth, fistulas and any infections that occur around the genital area and anus.

Antibiotics that may be prescribed include: **Ciprofloxacin (Cipro)** and **Metronidazole (Flagyl)**.

There are various side effects including:

With **Metronidazole (Flagyl)**:
- Diarrhea.
- Dizziness.
- Headaches.
- Loss of appetite.
- Nausea.
- Vomiting.

Note! Over a period of time this drug can cause a condition of neuropathy—a nervous disorder which causes tingling in the hands and feet.

With **Ciprofloxacin (Cipro)**:
- Interacts adversely if taken at the same time as antacids such as Rolaids and Tums.
- Interacts adversely if taken at the same time as calcium, iron or zinc in vitamin and mineral supplements.

Note! Therefore, do not take your dose of **Ciprofloxacin (Cipro)** at the same time as your antacids or vitamin and mineral supplements.

Anti-diarrhea drugs such as **Loperamide (Imodium)** or a combination of **Atropine** and **Diphenoxylate (lomotil)** may prove effective. Also **Codeine** may be prescribed in some cases.

I think this is the most depressing chapter in the entire book. Reading all the side effects makes one realize why so many people decide to try a more natural (alternative) route.

Chapter 13

Massage & Natural Ways to Help Control Crohn's Disease

Approximate estimates of the American population show that there are 100 out of every 100,000 who have been diagnosed with either ulcerative colitis or Crohn's disease. In many cases, physicians prescribe steroids, antibiotics and other opioids to help control the pain and inflammation.

However, some patients without medical insurance are unable to afford the medications, whilst others have an aversion to taking medication and prefer to try an alternative route.

Depending upon the severity of the disease, some alternative therapies can be very effective. Massage therapy is very effective for those suffering from Crohn's disease.

While Crohn's disease is not caused by stress, it can aggravate symptoms of the disease. In addition, stress can also aggravate many other conditions including: asthma, arthritis, lupus and heart disease.

Having massage therapy is not a cure for Crohn's disease; rather it provides relief from stress. Other avenues to explore to relieve stress include: yoga, meditation, exercise and consulting a naturopathic doctor who may suggest various naturopathic medicines. It is important though to ensure that the naturopathic doctor is properly licensed by the state that he or she is practicing in.

Massage sessions should be done by a licensed therapist with at least several years experience. A good massage therapist should be able to incorporate aromatherapy, hot stone therapy and heat therapy. In addition he / she should have a strong pair of hands to help relieve the tension in your muscles, as well as releasing lactic acid which will enhance your relaxation and decrease the soreness in your muscles.

If your physician recommends massage therapy to relieve stress, it would be a good idea to check with your insurance company, as this may count towards your annual deductible. If it doesn't, then it will definitely count towards the amount you can deduct from your taxes above the standard 7 percent. Ask your accountant for advice, and ask your doctor for a written confirmation that massage therapy will be beneficial for your condition to help back up your insurance claim.

Additional natural things you can try to alleviate pain and help bring your Crohn's disease under control include: ceasing drinking coffee, tea and any caffeinated drinks; eliminate milk and milk products such as cheese and ice cream from your diet. You could also try stress relievers such as biofeedback, do breathing exercises and have psychotherapy sessions; and finally take an Omega-3 EPA supplement to help the healing process.

When your Crohn's disease is in remission, a low fat, high fiber diet will help provide your body with the nutrients it needs and it will also help with the remission process.

Chapter 14

Crohn's Disease and Natural Remedies

Natural remedies are a popular alternative for people who suffer from Crohn's disease, as it is a means to avoid medications and in addition, if the individual cannot afford the medications it is a good alternative pathway to follow. Following a natural route gives the body the best chance to heal itself which can result in less relapses.

As mentioned previously, there is no known cure for Crohn's disease, but natural alternatives to medications can play a positive role in a treatment program, with no side effects.

One thing that I have not mentioned so far is the issue of a parasitic infection, especially in the gastrointestinal tract (GI Tract). Parasites are often thought of as a Third World issue where hygiene standards are not as high as they are in the US and Europe. However, it is estimated that approximately one third of the population of the United States may be infected with parasites at any one time.

Children in particular are very susceptible to these types of infections; for one reason, that their immune systems are not yet fully developed, and in small children, they have the habit of putting everything into their mouth.

Pets–especially dogs and cats can be carriers of parasites; so it is important to wash your hands carefully after stroking a pet–and especially before eating a meal.

Some parasites are actually in the food you eat–and they are just waiting for you to under-cook the food so that they can survive the cooking process and get inside your body.

Parasites thrive in a toxic environment, and those individuals suffering from Crohn's disease are particularly susceptible to a parasitic invasion.

The "Western Diet" does not help either, which is very high in saturated fat, sugar and often artificial ingredients, and low in fiber and enzymes to break down the food. Because the body finds it difficult to digest this type of food, a toxic and un-digested food build-up can occur which is just what parasites need for their food source.

So two major priorities for dealing with Crohn's disease are: building up the immune system, and making sure that you do not have a parasite infection, and if you do, to make sure you eradicate it.

There are quite a few natural products which you can consider for eliminating parasites. Here are a few of them:

Parasites and Worms

Black Walnut

Black walnut is an excellent anti-parasitic herb, especially against worms. It also has a high iodine content, which is good for energy as it supports thyroid function.

Cloves

Cloves are a good natural parasite cleansing herb which can be obtained as a liquid, powder or in a capsule.

Colloidal Silver

Although not an herb, colloidal silver has many uses and has been found to be effective against many surface micro-organisms, viruses, protozoa, amoeba, fungi, parasites and yeasts.

There are many different colloidal silver products on the market. You need to source one that contains 99.9 percent pure silver without any additives.

Grapefruit Seed Extract

Grapefruit seed extract is an effective anti-parasitic herb which has a very bitter taste. This can be sweetened by adding a small amount of honey.

Garlic

Garlic has so many uses from using it in cooking to it being an excellent product for heart health. It also has antibacterial, anti-fungus and antiviral properties. Other recognized health benefits of garlic, include acting as an antibiotic as well as other health advantages like its anti-cholesterol and anti-hypertensive properties.

It is also an antioxidant which protects the body against the effects of free radical damage. Its high sulfur content assists in cell purification.

Allicin is the principle biological active compound which gives garlic its odor. Be warned. Many so called "odorless" garlic products have the active compound removed which makes it rather worthless. It can be obtained as a garlic bulb, in a capsule or in tablet form.

Pumpkin Seeds

One of the best tasting of all the anti-parasite herbal products. The seeds can be eaten as a snack. In fact they taste so good that you cannot eat enough of them. Pumpkin seeds are very effective against tapeworms as well as other types of parasites. They also serve as a good source of essential fatty acids (EFAs) which are essential for good health.

(If you need further information on parasites my Book "*An easy way to understand parasites, worms, candida, constipation and detoxing*" is available as a print edition or for the Kindle platform on Amazon.com, or on the other Amazon country sites. It is also available for the Barnes and Noble "Nook".

Suggested Nutritional Supplements

Digestive Enzymes

Usually available in an enteric coated capsule form (enteric coated meaning the capsule is designed to dissolve in a part of the body where it is needed); these are important for breaking down undigested protein, so it can be more easily assimilated, and for dealing with toxins and parasites, so they can be eliminated. All of this will take a burden off the immune system.

Acidophilus

A probiotic supplement which is available in capsule form. It assists the body in replenishing friendly bacteria in the bowel, in addition to protecting against un-friendly bacteria. In addition, it assists the body to digest food, and in the healing process.

Live Yogurt

Live yogurt will help enhance friendly bacteria, especially if part of the small intestine has been removed. Alternatively, you can take a probiotic supplement containing lactobacillus bacteria.

Herbal and Miscellaneous Products

Aloe Vera Juice

Helps to keep the colon clean and assists in healing adhesions. Enhances digestion and reduces inflammation. It is also very soothing.

Bentonite Clay or Charcoal

Soaks up toxins and can stop diarrhea. It will also help purge any parasitic infestations.

Blue-Green Algae

Rich in minerals; blue-green algae has a cleansing action and assists in healing the digestive tract.

Chlorophyll

Rich in minerals; chlorophyll has a cleansing action and assists in healing the digestive tract.

Capsicum
Helps reduce inflammation and is used for healing internal bleeding.

Cats Claw (Una De Gato)
Has anti-inflammatory properties in addition to assisting in the healing process. It is excellent for cleansing the intestinal tract.

Co-Q10
Assists in healing damaged tissue and supports the immune system.

Germanium
Assists in healing damaged tissue and supports the immune system.

Goldenseal
Helps reduce inflammation and is used for healing internal bleeding

Licorice Root
Good for healing the digestive tract. Has anti-viral properties, and supports the adrenal glands during times of stress.

Marshmallow
Has a high mucilage content which is very soothing and healing to inflamed tissue.

Peppermint Oil
Available as a liquid and enteric coated capsules; peppermint oil has been found to reduce the inflammatory effects and symptoms of Crohn's disease. It relaxes the gastrointestinal smooth muscle.

Red Clover
A good blood cleanser in addition to it being a healer of the digestive tract.

Slippery Elm
Slippery Elm is very soothing to inflamed membranes. It also helps to control diarrhea.

Superoxide Dismutase (SOD)
SOD is an enzyme and free radical scavenger as well as a very effective antioxidant. As it helps to reduce the damaging effects of inflammatory conditions in the bowel, it has been used successfully to treat Crohn's disease.

Supplements for the Nervous System

Hops
A common aid for calming and relaxing the nerves. In fact, the nervous system is very sensitive to the health of the thyroid gland. Hops are widely used for insomnia or restless sleep, in addition to being a good source of

plant calcium; hops are also very effective for menstrual pain and muscle cramps.

Passion Flower

Acts as a mild sedative and is widely used for conditions of anxiety, hyperactivity in children, hypertension, irritability and nervous tension. In addition, it is very effective for nervous tension associated with PMT and nervous over-activity and panic. It has analgesic properties which help relieve menstrual pain, headaches and toothache.

St. John's Wort

St John's Wort is usually mentioned in any discussion relating to stress management or mild depression. In fact it has been used for centuries for these purposes. It contains the chemical compound hypericin. St John's Wort prevents the up-take of serotonin–a hormone, also called 5-hydroxytryptamine, found in the pineal gland, blood platelets, digestive tract, and the brain.

Serotonin actions are as a chemical messenger that passes nerve signals between nerve cells. When changes occur in brain levels of serotonin, this affects a person's mood and feeling of well-being. This is where St John's Wort comes in–like medications that affect the actions of serotonin which are used in the treatment of depression.

Valerian

Valerian Root—a natural plant calcium, is often used as a pain killer. It has been used for centuries to treat anxiety and insomnia. It relaxes muscle spasms associated with muscle and stomach cramp, and is best taken before bedtime.

Calcium

Sufficient calcium is essential for good nervous system health. It should be taken along with magnesium and vitamin D. Magnesium is often lacking in people who have Crohn's disease and is needed along with vitamin D for the absorption of calcium.

Vitamins and Minerals

It has long been established that you do not get all your daily requirements of vitamins and minerals from the food you eat. This is due to the way crops are grown, the way they are processed and finally how the food that is derived from those crops is prepared in the home. In addition to that, intensive farming methods over the years have depleted the minerals in the soil to such an extent that hardly any exist anymore. So I am going to continue this section with vitamin and mineral supplements rather than giving you a list of various foods that various vitamins and minerals can be obtained from.

Let me start with a multivitamin and multi-mineral supplement. There are plenty of them available in health food stores, by mail order and on-line. But what are they and what do they do?

Basically, they are designed to take care of any vitamin and mineral shortfall in your diet. If you look at the label you will usually see about 16 different vitamins and minerals listed. Some will have a RDA (recommended daily allowance) figure quoted as well–provided an RDA has been established by your government.

If your body has a shortfall in any particular vitamin and mineral, then it will take it from the supplement. If there is no deficiency, then the supplement will pass out harmlessly in the urine. So it is basically an insurance policy.

Another thing to bear in mind is that all vitamin and mineral supplements are not created equal. There are synthetic ones as well as natural ones. The synthetic ones are usually by-products of the petroleum industry, while natural ones are derived from plant sources. It is best if you purchase natural ones. They may be a little more expensive, but they do contain "live" ingredients which will nourish the body, as opposed to synthetic ones which are basically inert substances which are "dead".

So, here is a list of various vitamin and mineral supplements which may be beneficial to you in coping with the symptoms of Crohn's disease.

Vitamin A

Often taken as Beta Carotene which is converted to vitamin A by the liver as required. Vitamin A helps to heal the mucus membranes of the bowel as well as being important for proper metabolism of the intestinal mucosa. Encouraging clinical trials have shown that Vitamin A supplementation may be a successful treatment for Crohn's disease.

Vitamin B (Complex)

Like vitamin C, the B vitamins are water soluble and therefore are often depleted from the body during periods of stress. The B vitamins are needed to counteract nervous disorders and depressive tendencies. They are also needed to purge toxins and bad estrogen from the liver. All the B vitamins work together therefore it is best to take your B vitamins in a complex form. However, if you need individual B vitamins for some reason, then it is best to take them in addition to a B Complex supplement.

Vitamin C with Bioflavonoids

Vitamin C is a water soluble vitamin that is often depleted from the body during periods of stress. Bioflavonoid Compounds in vitamin C such as quercetin assist in inhibiting inflammatory responses in the intestines.

Vitamin D

Known as the sunshine vitamin due to it being synthesized through the skin by the actions of sunlight. People who suffer from chronic colon disorders are often deficient in this vitamin, therefore supplementation is essential. Vitamin D is needed for the absorption of calcium; therefore a lack of this vitamin can lead to a loss of calcium from the bones.

Vitamin E

An important free radical scavenger and antioxidant, vitamin E is important for healing tissue in the intestinal lining. Various studies have shown a substantial improvement when used as vitamin therapy for ulcerative colitis.

Vitamin K

Vitamin K is essential for blood clotting. In studies people who received vitamin K supplements showed an improvement in their Crohn's disease symptoms. Like vitamin D, people who suffer from chronic colon disorders are often lacking in vitamin K.

Folic Acid (Vitamin B9)

A folic acid deficiency is common in people suffering from Crohn's disease. It helps reduce the diarrhea associated with this disease.

Magnesium

As explained elsewhere, magnesium works with calcium and vitamin D. A deficiency of magnesium is common with individuals suffering from Crohn's disease.

Zinc

An antioxidant mineral. A deficiency has been identified in nearly 50 percent of people suffering from Crohn's disease.

Essential Fatty Acids

Both Omega-3 and Omega 6 essential fatty acids must be obtained from the diet–they cannot be made by the body. Good sources of EFA's are oily fish such as: salmon, mackerel, sardines and tuna. You can also take essential fatty acid supplements in capsule form. Essential fatty acids help reduce inflammation by elevating the production of prostaglandins which can be impaired in Crohn's disease.

Fiber Supplements

One of the biggest problems is that Americans do not get enough fiber in their diet. This is due to dietary choices made by individuals where the average diet is very high in fat, sugar and sodium (salt) and is also often highly processed. There are many forms of fiber available, from cereals to fiber supplements.

Probably bran is often thought of when fiber is considered, but be careful! Bran is a hard fiber and can irritate an already inflamed intestine. It contains a lot of phytic acid a compound that can block the uptake of many minerals including: calcium, magnesium, iron, zinc and copper to name a few. This may lead to a mineral deficiency at a later stage which can cause other problems such as osteoporosis. An iron deficiency can cause anemia.

Oats are a useful alternative to bran. For some reason wheat can irritate an inflamed intestine. Think more of a water soluble fiber or psyllium, both of which have proved effective for individuals suffering from diarrhea, pain and constipation. Fiber mixed with the herbs astragalus and schizandra are especially beneficial. Fiber is also good for cleansing and providing nourishment to the lower bowel. It is Important to drink plenty of water when taking any fiber supplement–ideally 6-8 glasses each day.

Protein

The usual sources of protein are red and white meat and fish. Red meat can be especially irritating to inflamed tissue and should be avoided. The outer skin should be removed from white meat (chicken and turkey etc). White fish is a good source of protein and oily fish mentioned earlier are a good source of essential fatty acids.

You could also consider a protein supplement. The three most common are whey, tofu and soy. Whey protein should be avoided as it is a by-product of cheese production.

Tofu is safe as it is derived from soy milk and is available in either blocks of tofu or in a powder form. Tofu is an Asian food and therefore can be used in cooking, or if in powder form then it can be mixed with liquid or a fiber supplement or cereals.

Soy protein is safe and is usually available in powder form which can be mixed with various juices in addition to water. It can also be mixed in with a fiber supplement or cereals.

Dietary Guidelines

- It is important to take vitamin and mineral supplements daily.
- Learn which foods cause irritation and pain and avoid them.
- If diarrhea is severe then a liquid diet may be best for a few days until the diarrhea has subsided.
- Juice fasting will be beneficial by taking pressure off the digestive system, in addition to supplying nutrients and helping with healing the GI tract.
- You could try carrot juice, cabbage juice, green juices and herbal teas. They are all rich in minerals and are beneficial.
- Try the following two juice mixtures which have healing properties. Mixture 1. Carrot, cabbage, parsley and ginger. Mixture 2. Carrot, celery, endive and garlic.
- Digestive enzymes are important. They will help to break down undigested protein, toxins and help eliminate parasites.
- Chew solid food thoroughly and avoid liquid drinks with meals.
- When a flare-up occurs, avoid food containing high roughage especially those that contain skins and seeds. It is a good idea to avoid popcorn.
- Vegetable soups are nourishing and healing. They are also rich in minerals. Always remember that minerals are vital. The body does not manufacture them–they must be obtained from the diet.
- Adding garlic and ginger to your soups will help kill any parasites and it will also help the healing process.
- You need potassium for good digestion, and this mineral is often compromised by an inflamed colon.
- You can also puree cooked vegetables which will make them easier on your digestive system, especially if you are experiencing a flare-up.
- Avoid dairy products.
- Avoid smoking which can irritate the GI tract.
- Avoid alcohol which can generate gas and as a result, can cause pain.
- Avoid fried foods as well as junk foods which can aggravate an inflamed condition.
- Foods to avoid include: coffee, tea, eggs, wheat gluten, and raw vegetables. Remember to remove the skin from chicken and turkey. Excessive red meat consumption increases bowel transit time with the result that the GI tract is not properly cleaned.

This is a long chapter but I felt it was important to give you some options and information that I hope will be helpful in getting your Crohn's disease into remission and keeping it there. I have always personally preferred the natural route as it is healthier and side effects are dramatically reduced or eliminated. Always remember to keep a record of any foods that cause Crohn's disease to flare-up and you will then know to avoid them in the future.

By being cautious about what you eat and drink, you can lead a full life and be in control of this disease rather than the disease being in control of you.

Please note! I have not included any contraindications in this chapter as to how natural remedies may interact with any medications you may have been prescribed. Every case is different so it is important that you consult your physician or a naturopathic doctor before you start taking any natural products as your medication may need adjustment, or you may be advised that a particular product featured in this chapter is unsuitable for you.

Chapter 15

In Summary

Crohn's disease was renamed in 1932 from ileitis. It was named after Burrill Bernard Crohn. It is an inflammatory bowel disease along with ulcerative colitis. Crohn's disease can cause inflammation in any area of the digestive tract from the mouth to the anus. However, most instances occur in the large and small intestines.

- It is still unknown what causes Crohn's disease.
- Various factors can increase the risk.
- The common age range is between 20–30 years, but it can be diagnosed in children and older adults.
- Crohn's disease appears to be associated mainly with Western countries where the diet is poor, the lifestyle is fast and there are excessive stress factors.
- Some physicians believe that Crohn's disease is an autoimmune disease where the body attacks its own cells causing inflammation.
- Black Americans are at a lower risk of developing Crohn's disease.
- Jewish people have a higher risk of developing the disease.
- Although there is no cure, there are ways to control the disease and keep it in a remissive state.
- Crohn's disease is not contagious.
- There may be some genetic link as approximately 20 percent of those diagnosed with Crohn's disease have a close blood relative who also has the disease.
- There are equal numbers of men and women who are affected.
- There are approximately 2 millions Americans diagnosed with the disease and approximately 95,000 in the UK. Roughly 1 out of every 600 people.
- The most common symptoms are diarrhea and abdominal pain.
- Additional symptoms may include: arthritis, inflammation of the eye, fever, skin disorders, weight loss and rectal bleeding.
- There are various treatment options currently available including: dietary and lifestyle changes, surgery, drugs and nutritional supplements.
- The main purpose is to control inflammation, ease symptoms and keep the disease in remission.
- Complications can include: abscesses, obstructions, narrowing and perforation in the intestines, stomach distention, ulcers, scarring, feelings of nausea and vomiting.

- It is important to stop smoking and drink only small amounts of alcohol–if any at all.
- Improve the nutritional intake and avoid foods that cause a relapse.
- If the disease is in remission, don't take chances by eating foods that you know have caused a relapse in the past. In remission, you may feel well, but the disease is not cured—it is always there!
- Remember to consult your doctor or a naturopathic doctor before changing your diet, or commencing taking vitamin, mineral or herbal supplements, as these may interfere with any medication that you may be taking.

About The Author

Brian B Jacques has been a natural health researcher for over thirty years. He has presented seminars worldwide on such diverse subjects as Health Related issues, Motivation and Personal Development. In addition he has written numerous books, newsletters and articles on these subjects.

His very popular Series of Mini-Health Books includes:

- An Easy Way To Understand Eczema and Psoriasis
- An Easy Way To Understand Stress and Depression
- Amino Acids & Enzymes—What Are They & Why Do You Need Them
- An Easy Way To Understand Vitamins and Minerals
- An Easy Way To Understand Crohn's Disease and IBD
- An Easy Way To Understand Body Building For Men And Women
- An Easy Way To Understand Alzheimer's Disease
- An Easy Way To Understand Herpes
- An Easy Way To Understand Parkinson's Disease
- An Easy Way To Understand Autism
- An Easy Way To Understand Fibromyalgia
- The Little A–Z Dictionary of Herbal Remedies
- Effective Methods To Stop Smoking
- The Magic Of Vitamins & Minerals
- An Easy Way To Understand Your Body Systems
- An Easy Way To Understand Erectile Dysfunction
- An Easy Way To Understand Heart Disease, High Blood Pressure & Stroke
- An Easy Way To Understand Detoxing For Men & Women
- How To Lose Weight After 40
- How To Lose Weight And Maintain Your Ideal Weight Permanently

All these books are available as Kindle Editions (available from the Kindle Store on Amazon.com, and other countries Amazon sites where the Kindle platform is supported.) Many of these books are also available for the Barnes and Noble "Nook". In addition, all these titles will shortly be available as print editions from the Amazon website.

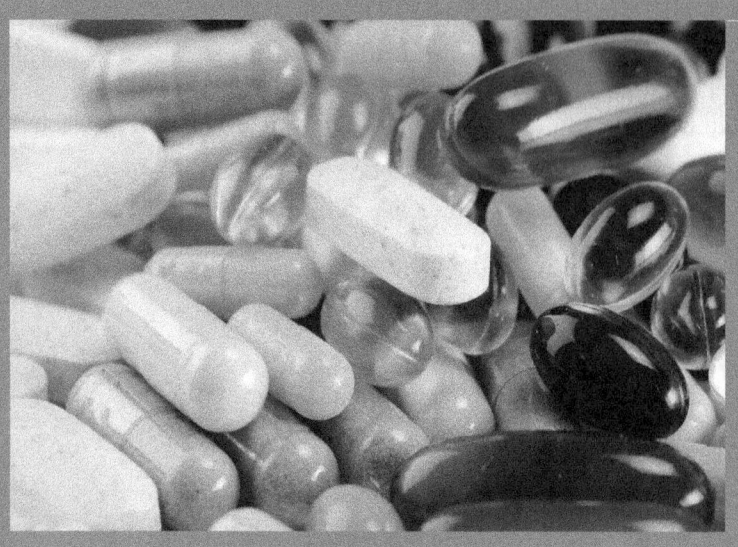

Index

Brian B Jacques.